The 28 Day DASH DIET

WEIGHT-LOSS PROGRAM:
Simple Steps To Transform Your
Body In 28 Days

N. Valorous

Copyright © 2024

Disclaimer

You are encouraged to print this book for easy reading.

Table of Contents

Introduction
You're Not Alone

Welcome to "The 28-Day Dash Diet".

Before we begin, there are a few important things to mention. Losing weight is a mind game. If you change your mind, you'll change your body. It's inevitable.

When we say "change your mind," we don't mean changing your mind from eating cookies to devouring cake.

What we're talking about here is the mindset behind any weight loss. It doesn't matter your age or gender. The principles are the same.

First, you need to stop hating your body. Far too many women think poorly of themselves. They feel that they're fat and ugly while all the other women are better.

Maybe you've been wanting to have a "thigh gap," but you can't even find clothes that fit you at The Gap.

"Why can't I look like her?". "It sucks being me!" "I have horrible fatty genes!"

These are just some ways women beat themselves up. Here's the truth...You need to love yourself for what you are,

flab, rolls, cellulite, and all.

This weight loss journey has to begin with self-love for you.

You will continue to struggle with bad self-image even after you lose weight if you don't alter this mentality.You will never be good enough for you.

Accept yourself. And from there you can improve. This is a journey and not an overnight miracle.

Look in the mirror. That's your competition. Not anyone else.

You should also understand that you can lose weight. By assuming that you have 'fat genes' or that it's more difficult for you to lose weight, you make it a self-fulfilling prophecy.

There will be times when you slip up. This is inevitable and par for the course. When striving for a noble goal, the journey is never linear.

It's often fraught with minor setbacks, slip-ups, mistakes, etc. What you need to understand is that every setback is a setup for a comeback.

During those times, if you slip up on your diet, don't just be weak and give up just because you made one mistake in your diet.

Don't punish yourself if you have a piece of cake after work and then eat everything that falls into your mouth the rest of the day. Recognize your error and try to avoid it in the future.

This one tiny mistake won't matter if you stay on course for the following few days. You can be sure that the weight will come back on if you give up on your diet and abandon it.

You are not your mistake. Acknowledge, correct it, and avoid future mistakes and KEEP MOVING. That is the only way to succeed.

You're definitely in control of your body and can change for the better if you know what to do. This book will tell you what you should do.

All that you need to do is follow it to the letter and you will reach your desired weight. By doing so, you will gain energy, become stronger, feel happy, and have an indescribable sense of accomplishment.

Does that excite you? It should!

Read on.

Chapter 1
The Struggle Is Real

Yes, it is.

This is what the weight loss companies and diet pill manufacturers don't want you to know. Weight loss is a hard process.
The concept is brain-dead simple. All you need to do is burn more calories than you consume. That's all it is. If you remove all the fluff and hype, it always boils down to this one principle.
You need to eat the right foods in the right quantities and get sufficient exercise.
The diet pill companies will tell you that you can achieve staggering results–Lose 12 Pounds in 7 Days! Without starving yourself. Easy weight loss! That's always their angle. You can know by common sense that these medications are ineffective. After all, how can you lose weight by eating something else?

To convince you that these pills work, the supplement companies will list a bunch of ingredients that sound exotic and supposedly have fat-burning properties. Because the truth is a tough pill to swallow, women fall for this propaganda. It's challenging to exercise and clean up your nutrition. Taking weight loss pills is easy.
And everybody wants it easy.
Easy things often lead to disappointment, regret, and a loss of time and money. This is a heavy price to pay most often, you'll never see any results.
That's why you see women going from pill to pill. This explains why there are constantly new weight loss products available.
 When people realize that it's not working, they try the next product and the next, and this vicious cycle doesn't end.
You need to understand that most of the time; you gain weight gradually. Nobody wakes up 20 pounds heavier overnight. Your body got fatter over time.

To lose the fat, it will take time. This book emphasizes that you'll transform your body in 28 days, and it will. If you do what it says. He doesn't make wild promises to lose 20 pounds a week. In the best-case scenario, you might lose 3 to 4 pounds a week, and you'll lose about 12 or maybe 8 pounds in 4 weeks.

It all depends on your body, the more excess weight you have, the more weight you will lose. It's a strange contradiction, but larger people lose weight faster.

The more weight you lose, the more difficult it becomes.

Whatever the case may be, 28 days is a good time frame to aim for. You will see the difference

In the fitness sector, there is a quote.

It takes 4-week for you to see your body changing.

It requires eight weeks for your relatives and friends.

For the rest of the world, it takes 12 weeks.

KEEP GOING

This is very true. In 28 days, the transformation you'll see will motivate you to keep going because you know that what you're doing works.

Most give up when they don't see results quickly enough.

Usually, they've just not given themselves enough time.

You'll need to plan your weight loss, then you'll realize just how long it will take you to reach your goal. We'll be looking at this in the next chapter.

The important part of it is that it keeps things realistic for you. If you're looking at 8 weeks to reach your dream body, you won't lose motivation and give up after two weeks because you have six more weeks to go.

You also will not believe the hype the infomercials and supplements throw at you.

Your body works at its own pace. It's not affected by hype fantasies, or weight loss based on natural laws. You wear what you eat. You need to move more and need to stay on the course. This is what transforms your body.

It doesn't sound glamorous or fun, but the truth seldom does.

Nevertheless, you can lose weight. You ALWAYS can. Now let's move on to the next chapter where I show you how long it takes you to reach your desired weight.

Chapter 2
Planning & Tracking Your Progress

Finding out what your daily caloric deficit should be is the first thing you should do.

HERE ARE WHAT WE'RE GOING TO COVER IN THIS CHAPTER

1. How to track weight loss progress

2. Don't forget to track your feelings

There is no dispute: losing weight requires more effort. However, that does not preclude having a little fun.

Discovering fun methods to monitor your progress might be a thrilling aspect of your weight loss journey, as weight loss is a gradual process. There are more options than ever before to help you stay on course today.

Here are seven ways to track weight loss. Observe and consider what might work for you.

1. Use a scale

This option has a proven track record for a reason. When choosing a bathroom scale, read reviews to see if others found it provided an accurate reading. Studies show that digital home bathroom scales offer more precise readings than those old analog scales.

If you can, weigh yourself on a scale multiple times at the store.

If it gives you the same number each time, it's a keeper.

Remember: fluctuations in body weight are normal. If exercise is part of your routine, don't fret if your weight plateaus or even goes up a bit. As you burn fat and increase muscle mass, your weight typically increases. That's because muscle weighs more than fat.

Remember that weight is only a number as well.

If you could snap your fingers and be your ideal size, would the number on the scale matter? Probably not. That said, a scale can help you keep track of your progress by reaching your goals.

Make an effort to weigh yourself every day, ideally just after you urinate in the morning. When you do it, wear the same item of clothing or nothing at all. You'll get the most accurate reading this way.

Keep a log on your phone to monitor your progress, but don't let little shifts in the other direction get you down.

2. Monitor your BMI

Your BMI, or body mass index, is a ratio of weight and height. More specifically, it's your weight in kilograms divided by your height in meters squared. A healthy BMI for adults is typically between 18.5–24.9 kg/m2.

Yes, we know, it's a little messy to calculate (though there are plenty of online calculators to do the math for you). While BMI seems to be a favorite among healthcare providers for tracking weight, it might not be the best option.

That's because it doesn't do a great job of accounting for the variability in body composition. Take, for example, a bodybuilder. Medium height, tons of muscle, and not an ounce of fat on their body, yet their BMI will be through the roof—even looking unhealthy according to clinical standards.

Why? Because the calculation doesn't consider the person or their body composition. It just looks at height and weight. It misses crucial factors by lumping everyone into one large bucket, such as the fact that women frequently have higher body fat than males and that physically active persons have lower body fat.

body fat than non-active individuals and older people often have more body fat than those younger.

Since this measure isn't a great one, it's unlikely a healthcare provider will prescribe any sort of intervention based on BMI alone. That said, it can still serve as a rough estimate of weight loss—as long as you take your results with a grain of salt.

3. Bust out the tape measure

Measuring your body can be a useful tool for monitoring weight loss regardless of whether you're on a certain diet, doing regular exercise, or a combination of the two.

Additionally, monitoring your body's measurements can occasionally indicate your general health.

Higher body weight and larger circumferences (particularly in the chest and waist) are associated with health issues like diabetes, and heart disease, and of course, these measurements are not an exact science. To assess your risk of developing these conditions, your healthcare provider can perform tests and make recommendations based on the results.

Take regular measures of your chest, waist, hips, thighs, calves, upper arms, and forearms to monitor your progress in losing weight.

4. Notice how your clothes fit

That's right. As simple as getting dressed will assist you in keeping an eye on your weight. One clothing size equals roughly 10–15 pounds, so you can track your weight loss journey simply by noticing when it's time to buy new clothes.

5. Take a selfie

Taking photos can help you see how far you've come, and provides evidence to keep you motivated on days when you're feeling stuck.

It takes time to see weight loss, so you don't need to take a photo every day. Instead, take one every few weeks or once a month. To make it easier to see results, take a selfie from the same angle each time and wear the same type of outfit.

6. Use a weight tracking app

You know there's an app for that! Monitor Your Weight (available on iOS and Android) is a top-rated option.

You can also track body weight using your smartphone's built-in health app, or buy a smart scale that automatically communicates that information to your phone.

Smart scales have the added benefit of measuring more than just body weight. They also estimate body fat percentage, muscle mass, and bone mass to give you a more holistic picture of your health.

7. Be consistent in your tracking

Our body weight fluctuates throughout the day and week. There are many contributing factors to this, including when you eat, drink, exercise, get dressed, or even go to the bathroom.

Make sure you're comparing apples to apples to prevent manipulating the figures and any resulting disappointment.

This means taking your measurements on the same day each week. If you dare, go bare. If not, dress uniformly for every reading to ensure consistency.

Remember to monitor your emotions.

For whatever reason, you're keeping a weight diary to change for the better.

So, this should be a positive experience.

For some people, monitoring keeps them on track toward their weight loss goals. For others, it causes needless tension and has a detrimental effect on their mental well-being.

Know what works for you so you can stay positive about your weight loss journey.

Chapter 3
Mastering Hunger & Conquering Emotional Overeating

Let's face it. You will need to eat less if you wish to reduce your weight. Indeed.

You don't want to. You enjoy eating. Do you have to cut down your calorie intake?

Yes.

What if you eat the same amount and just exercise? No. Eating less is still necessary.

Ok. You'll eat the same amount, exercise like crazy, and pop a few slimming pills too. Is that ok? No. You'll still have to eat less.

Now that we have established that fact, we can move on. It is not the case that we should eat like birds when we advocate for eating less. You'll never run out of food to keep yourself nourished, robust, and in good health.

The problem society faces these days is that people eat too much. They eat when they're happy. They eat when they're sad.

For fear of going without food later, people eat when they are hungry and when they are not.

Once you aim to cut your calories, you will end up eating less than you're accustomed to. Since you're already in the habit of eating a certain quantity of food daily, the body is going to feel a little hungry.

This is normal. You're not starving. Your body needs time to adjust to the fewer calories. There will be slight discomfort and you may find yourself thinking of food often. You will need to exercise willpower and not eat. Reducing weight requires maintaining a calorie deficit.

Look at it as a challenge that you can surmount. Many women look at controlling their diet as an enormous pain in the butt.

There are 7 tips in this chapter to curb your appetite. These will help to a certain extent to control your cravings. Please take note that your hunger will naturally decrease after a week of maintaining a caloric deficit.

You'll want to eat less the less you consume. You'll need less food to feel full because your stomach will get smaller.

It can take a week or two for that to occur. Your daily food intake will determine how long it takes, but be assured that you will require less food as you progress.

7 Tips for Curbing Hunger

Skip breakfast.

This contradicts all you have heard thus far. On the other hand, research indicates that eating your first meal later in the day will result in reduced overall food consumption. Go ahead and have breakfast if you really must, but make sure it's light and high in protein. Leave off the white bread and sugary cereals.

Drink lots of water.

It'll make you feel full and very often people mistake thirst for hunger. You also need to be sufficiently hydrated to accelerate fat loss.

Consume a tablespoon or 2 of virgin coconut oil daily.

Studies have demonstrated that it decreases one's appetite, promotes leanness, and reduces the tendency to store fat.

Stay active throughout the day.

Sedentary activities such as vegetating in front of the TV for hours, playing video games non-stop, watching movies at the cinema, etc. will automatically make you want to pop something in your mouth to munch. Avoid these activities.

Eat lots of vegetables.

Vegetables such as broccoli, spinach, carrots, cauliflower, kale, celery, etc. contain a ton of beneficial properties. Not only are they good for your health, but they will also leave you feeling fuller for longer.

Use smaller plates.

This is a psychological trick. Smaller plates look fuller with less food. So, your brain automatically assumes you're eating a lot when you're not.

Go to bed earlier.

A bad habit that many people engage in is binge eating at night. This is usually because they're awake watching TV and end up feeling hungry. If you find that you're getting hungry at night, go to bed earlier. You will not struggle against cravings.

Follow the tips above and you will reduce the amount that you eat. Once you achieve this feat, your weight loss will go from being a possibility to a probability and, finally, a reality. Your success greatly depends on your nutrition. Never forget that.

Chapter 4
Do You Need To Diet?

Although you don't have to diet, you do need to stick to your plan.

Does that sound confusing?

Many women make the mistake of starving themselves, hoping to lose weight fast. This is counterproductive and works against them.

You need to be on a diet that is right for you, and most importantly, you need to be at a caloric deficit.

As long as you're at a caloric deficit, you will lose weight.

You're probably wondering. "What if I continued to have a caloric deficit even though I ate junk food?"

In theory, yes. It's not so simple, but yes.
You can lose weight even while eating fast
food, processed food, and junk food,
whatever they may call it. You know what
these foods are. C

As mentioned in Chapter 1, if you consume
fewer calories than your maintenance level,
you will lose weight.

Thus, in theory, you would lose weight even
if you consumed 500 calories less than your
maintenance level and went on a junk food
diet for the entire day.

Many overweight women almost always
have a very poor diet. It is extremely difficult
for them to switch from a diet that is so high
in processed/junk food to one that is clean
and wholesome.

It's only going to set you up for failure to
expect to change your diet completely
overnight.

You absolutely must do this slowly and progressively. Therefore, your best course of action will be to carry on eating the way you have but aim for a caloric deficit.

This basically means that you won't be eating as much junk food as you formerly did.
This in itself will help you lose weight.

However, since the goal is to lose weight and get healthy, your end goal should be to eliminate junk food from your diet and eat clean.

Every week, make one small positive change to your diet. You could swap up your typical lunch of two cheeseburgers and a Coke for a crispy tuna wrap and a glass of chilled coconut water.

Psychologically, this is easier. It's just one meal. Keep at it till this becomes a habit and you slowly but surely replace all the junk meals with wholesome yet tasty meals.

Healthy meals can be delicious too. You are not sacrificing taste or pleasure by eating healthily. It's just a matter of getting your taste buds and body to enjoy eating healthy foods, it can be accomplished over time.

You can maintain a calorie deficit while eating junk food and yet lose weight in the interim.

It's also important to remember that junk food lacks nutrients. This implies that you can be consuming junk food and yet feel hungry a short while later. This is a result of your body not having enough nutrition. This is one of the reasons why, even with a healthy diet, you will always feel hungry.

Also, note that certain processes within the body will prevent you from losing weight beyond a certain point. The body is a highly complex organism. It will lose weight for a while since you are in a caloric deficit. But over time, you'll find it harder and harder to do so.

Calorie intake must be less than calorie expenditure, however this is not just a mathematical equation. There are further variables, such as the caliber of the calories ingested and the food's thermogenic effect.

So, ideally, you may consume junk food at a caloric deficit, and over a month or two, slowly wean yourself off these unhealthy foods and get on a healthy diet.

Of course, you may indulge in junk food once in a while. Many of those who have switched, meanwhile, report that they never again feel the need to eat junk food.

Eating meals that promote fat burning is one of the best strategies to reduce weight through diet.

You'll feel fuller and your body will burn more calories if you include these foods in your diet. Unlike weight loss supplements, these foods work. And they're cheaper.

Foods That Burn Fat

Almonds

Oatmeal

Eggs

Legumes & Beans

Berries

Olive oil

Green vegetables

Lean meats and oily fish

Green tea

Avocadoes

All-natural peanut butter

You can reduce your appetite and speed up the burning of fat just by eating these items.

So, while you do not need to follow a highly restricted diet and starve yourself, you should aim to consume foods that are beneficial to your health.

You'll be amazed at just how much good food you can eat when it's not processed. We will examine the healthiest foods for you and the most effective weight loss strategy in the upcoming chapter.

Okay.

Chapter 5
Whole Foods and Wrong Foods.

Before telling you what the good foods to eat are, here is one of the BEST ways to lose weight fast.

Are you ready?

Cut Your Carbohydrate Intake and Processed Foods!

Carbohydrate intake is one of the biggest factors affecting the speed at which you lose weight. The main reason most women gain weight is that they consume too much processed carbs.

Processed carbohydrates, such those found in pasta, donuts, white bread, and potatoes, provide the body with a lot of fuel and calories quickly accumulate.

It shuttles all the excess fuel into its fat stores, and that's how you gain weight. Also, processed carbs usually cause a spike in insulin levels, which indirectly leads to weight gain. A double whammy.

The fact is that a restricted carb intake will do wonders for your fat loss. Studies have shown that restricting your carbs is more effective than restricting your calories.

So, if you are on a 500-calorie deficit daily, and your carb intake is minimal, you will lose much more weight in the same period than you would by consuming carbs while on a deficit.

Does that make sense? In simple words, fewer carbs equals more fat loss. Sounds good? You bet!

When you cut down your carb intake, your body will burn more fat from its fat stores because it doesn't have much carbs to burn for fuel. So, fat loss is faster.

Your body's blood sugar level will drop and people with diabetes will see an improvement in their condition. A restrictive carb diet also keeps type 2 diabetes at bay since your body's insulin sensitivity is on point.

Your good cholesterol levels will go up and your bad cholesterol levels will drop. Many people assume that cholesterol is related to fat intake.
The truth is that a high carb intake also hurts your cholesterol levels. Studies reveal that, in contrast to popular opinion, a low-carb diet lowers triglycerides more effectively than a low-fat diet.
It is crucial to remember that you should never go overboard. This also holds true for carb limitation.
Certain diets, like the Atkins diet, focus on severely limiting carbohydrates for extended periods of time.
This is detrimental to your body because you will end up fatigued, moody, and weak. The diet is not sustainable and once you come off it, you will gain whatever weight you lost and a bit more.
Excessive carb restriction will compromise your immune system, lead to muscle loss, slow down your fat burning, and put you in a weight loss plateau.

Your body's testosterone production will fall, and you will have a suppressed thyroid output. You'll also develop leptin resistance, which doesn't bode well for fat loss.

So, what do you do? How do you strike the right balance? You want the best of both worlds, don't you?

The only way to achieve this is with a technique that is known as carb cycling. You will fast from carbs for periods ranging from three to six days.

If you are overweight and have a slower metabolism, you should aim for 5 to 6 days of minimal or zero carbs.

You only need to cut carbs for three or four days if you're trying to shed a few additional pounds.

After the period of carb restriction, you will follow it with one day of carb intake. This is known as your "refeed" day.

Consume sufficient carbs on this day and you will give your body the fuel that it needs.

Your body will experience an increase in energy when its fuel reserves are restored, which will also speed up your metabolism.

Stick to healthy carbs such as sweet potatoes, whole grain bread, whole grain pasta, etc. You should aim for a 500 to 700-calorie surplus over the maintenance level. This will put your body back in fat-burning mode.
Use this technique repeatedly to fast your fat loss and improve your health. The day will come when you won't crave for carbs or processed junk foods.
When your body becomes healthy, its taste will change. That's why fit people can constantly make wise food choices. The rest is simple once you've overcome the initial difficulty of giving up these foods.

Your insulin sensitivity will improve, the pounds will drop and you will look and feel like a brand new you.

There is a saying—"Your abs are made in the kitchen, not the gym." What that means is that almost 80% of your success at weight loss or getting lean depends on your diet. When it comes to weight loss, most of your attention must focus on your diet.

The following 7 foods will undermine any attempts you make to lose weight.
There is absolutely no doubt that you have everything to gain and nothing to lose by giving these foods a pass.
The problem is that many people love these comfort foods and hate giving them up.
Sugar is addictive.
The more sugary foods you eat, the more you'll crave. So, by eliminating them slowly, you'll slowly condition your body to crave these foods less and less.
The following 7 foods will undermine any attempts you make to lose weight.
There is absolutely no doubt that you have everything to gain and nothing to lose by giving these foods a pass.

The problem is that many people love these comfort foods and hate giving them up.
Sugar is addictive.
The more sugary foods you eat, the more you'll crave. So, by eliminating them slowly, you'll slowly condition your body to crave these foods less and less.
7 Foods You Should AVOID at All Costs! Doughnuts are probably one of the unhealthiest foods on the planet. They consist of nothing more than refined carbohydrates and sugar.
They are high in calories, fats, carbs, and other preservatives. Continued consumption of doughnuts will lead to weight gain and digestive problems.
Fast food. Enough said.
Chips are just about everybody's guilty pleasure. Oh, the pleasures of munching on them while the movie plays.
 Chips have high levels of trans fats because of the hydrogenated vegetable oils that are used to fry the chips. This will lead to weight gain and cardiovascular disease.

French fries. It has been said that French fries are more deadly than cigarettes. This might have some validity.

High in trans fats and carcinogens, these foods can cause cancer.

Bagels are another crowd-pleaser. It has a very high glycemic index. It causes insulin spikes, which creates inflammation in the body along with other health issues. Acne, body aches, clogged arteries, mood swings, etc. are all consequences of fluctuating insulin levels, along with weight gain naturally.

Don't eat the bagel in the morning. Forego the bagel in favor of a 30-minute stroll. That should give you a general notion of how harmful it is.

Microwave popcorn. All the rage these days. Convenient, tasty, and fun. Yet, they contain carcinogens and diacetyl. Both cause cancer.

Cereals are another fat gain culprit. Despite being advertised as "healthy natural foods,"

the majority of cereals are not healthy for you. Cereals are hardly naturally occurring. These are genetically engineered foods that, over time, may cause harm to you. Just staying away from bad meals is half the fight won.
Always remember the long-term effects. Don't give in to sinful pleasures in the short term, which may lead to suffering in the long run.
Important Foods You Should Eat.

Proteins

Dicing protein takes more energy than digesting fats or carbohydrates. This implies that digesting a 200-calorie steak piece could theoretically result in a 40-calorie burn. On the other hand, digesting an ice cream will require very few calories.
This implies that a significant portion of your daily calories have to come from foods high in protein. Legumes and meats are excellent providers of protein. If you are doing a

weight training regimen, the protein will also assist you in gaining muscle. Aim for about 0.8 grams per pound of body weight.

The protein will build more muscle. When you have more muscle, you end up burning more fat. This is a good cycle to be in. That's the reason you might have noticed that fit and strong people seem to be able to consume more. Their muscles are burning more calories around the clock.

Good sources of protein are skinless chicken, lean beef, tuna, sardines, chickpeas, eggs, and salmon. The fish contains Omega-3 fatty acids. They are therefore even more advantageous to the body.

Certain meals' chemical compositions set off bodily mechanisms that lead to fat loss. Thus, consuming these foods will awaken your body and increase fat burning.

Verdant Tea

Among them is green tea. Avoid using sugar. It tastes a little bad, but it gets the job done.

Other Foods
Chilies, lemons, oranges, mangoes, garlic, ginger, and onions are all foods that contain many powerful antioxidants and nutrients that strengthen your immune system. When you are strong, your workouts will be better and you will burn more fat.
When most women first start a weight loss program, one issue they frequently encounter is feeling hungry all the time.

Food is always on their mind, and it takes a toll on their willpower.

One way to prevent this is to consume foods that are high in fiber and digest slowly.
You'll experience sustained fullness.
Foods that are high in fiber are easily digested and passed through the digestive tract sooner. That means fewer calories are absorbed, resulting in less tendency to gain weight.
Consume foods like oatmeal, oats, brown rice, whole grain bread and broccoli.

Broccoli is so good for your body that you should make it a staple in your diet.
The goal here is to consume whole foods and not processed foods. Whole foods are typically located around the outside of stores.
You will be removing yourself from processed foods as long as you stay away from the food on the inner shelves and aisles.
Finally, despite the fact that these meals are very helpful, they won't aid in weight loss unless you follow a healthy exercise routine and are in a calorie deficit.

The 2 key components to any fat loss are a caloric deficit while on a balanced diet and a good exercise program. Everything else is just gravy.
So, no matter how good and clean your diet is, make sure you're still at a daily caloric deficit.

Chapter 6
Water Not Wine

Although having the occasional glass of wine is acceptable, when trying to reduce weight, you shouldn't drink water.

The easiest way to get fat is to drink your calories. Steer clear of sodas, fruit juices offered in stores, sports drinks, etc. You only need water!

And you should drink lots of it.

This is why you should drink water.

Your metabolism is accelerated in the morning when you drink ice-cold water.

Your appetite is diminished by it. Drink a glass or two of water whenever you feel like nibbling to feel full and reduce your likelihood of snacking.

It keeps you hydrated and healthy.

Your body needs water to metabolize fat.

It's part of the fat-burning process.

Regular water consumption will reduce the risk of dehydration during physical activity.

This doesn't need to be emphasized anymore. Drink enough water daily.

Chapter 7
The Power of Protein

One of the best methods for accelerating weight loss is this one.

The more proteins you consume, the faster you lose weight. Protein digestion requires the body to expend extra energy. Proteins burn more calories than fats and carbohydrates, which are quickly and easily absorbed.

Never consume a carb without protein. Never eat fat without first consuming protein.

Just by having the protein together with these foods, you'll prevent an insulin spike.

Eating eggs is one of the best methods to increase your protein intake.

Eggs are among the healthiest foods available. They have received a bad rep about high cholesterol and other false information.

It is quite odd that although eggs are genuinely good, people consider harmful cereals to one's health to be healthy.

This book will correct the misinformation. A significant source of protein, omega-3 fatty acids, and many other healthful nutrients are eggs.

Cholesterol in the body is because of saturated fat and trans fat and not dietary cholesterol. That means that despite what you have been told, eating the eggs with the yolk is just fine.

Since the yolk contains most of the nutrients, it is healthier.

Eggs are a significant source of heart-healthy omega-3 fatty acids and lean protein, but they also provide several other vital minerals.

Many consider eggs to be the ideal food. They contain vitamin D, 7 grams of protein, vitamins B6, B12, choline, leucine, L-arginine, and folate. You may not be familiar with what most of these vitamins are, but what really matters is that they are what your body truly needs.

What truly matters is how you prepare the eggs and that you consume them in moderation. Avoid frying eggs in vegetables or fatty fat. Use coconut oil or olive oil. Fry them lightly or half-boil them.

The point to note is that when you are losing weight, mix 2 egg yolks and the rest should be egg whites. This is assuming that you're having more than 2 eggs.

The reason for this is that egg yolks, though high in protein, are calorie-dense. So, you want the benefits that eggs provide, but you do not want to add too many calories to your diet.

If this doesn't convince you, studies from the Rochester Centre for Obesity in America showed that eating eggs for breakfast can reduce daily calorie intake by more than 400 calories. Isn't that fantastic?

One point to note is that if you consume eggs daily, you will get more than enough protein. It would be ideal to avoid protein shakes and other commercial protein products sold in your health stores. Ideally, we should be getting our proteins from natural sources.

Also, try to get organic eggs. They will contain fewer omega-6 fats and more omega-3 fats.

If you're a vegetarian and don't eat eggs. Many vegetables are high in protein too. You can eat those and achieve the same benefits.

20 High Protein Veggies

Peas (Green)

Mange Tout (Edible-Podded Peas, cooked)

Sweet Corn (Yellow)

Succotash (Corn And Limas, cooked)

Sprouted Beans, Peas & Lentils (Soybean Sprouts)

Lima Beans (Cooked)

Kale

Broccoli Raab (Cime di Rapa, cooked)

Parsley

Artichokes (Globe or French)

Spinach (Cooked)

Mushrooms (White, cooked)
Collard Greens
Mustard Greens
Broccoli
Baby Zucchini (Courgettes)
Garden Cress
Beet Greens (Cooked)
Arugula (Rocket)
Brussels Sprouts (Cooked).

Chapter 8
Sleep Your Way To Weight Loss

Sleeping sufficiently is essential for weight loss.

Insufficient sleep causes your body to become stressed out and release a hormone called cortisol. This hormone leads to weight gain indirectly.

What most people don't realize is that being constantly deprived of sleep will take a toll on your health in the long run.

Research has shown that people who have less sleep eat more, feel hungrier and generally consume 350 calories more than required. Those who stay awake late often find themselves eating snacks and heavy meals often.

Insulin sensitivity and glucose tolerance will decline in your body. This is detrimental since it will cause your body to store fat rather than burn it. You will store fat far more readily if your insulin sensitivity is low. The same applies to glucose tolerance.

Once more, the body's capacity to burn fat diminishes or, in the worst instance, ceases entirely.

Your body will be under constant stress if you are exercising every day and eating over calories. Sleep is necessary for it to recuperate and mend. In addition, de-stress.

There's a reason "beautiful sleep" is utilized.

If you can't afford to get enough sleep at night, it will hamper all the best attempts at losing weight. Power naps during the day will not cut it.

You need to sleep at night for at least 7 hours. Most claim to survive on less. They might, but it will eventually come at a cost to their health.

Try to increase your productivity so that you can complete more tasks at work and avoid having to remain late. Give up late-night TV and avoid working out just before bed. Ideally, you should do exercise during the day.

Try to meditate to help you decompress from the tensions of everyday life. Recall that you are still a rat even if you win the rat race. Life is not just about goals, deadlines, and evaluations.

It will be much easier for you to lose weight if you get enough sleep. Getting enough sleep is of great significance and should never be undervalued.

Make sure you receive between 6 and 8 hours of sleep every day. While trying to

lose weight, don't burn the candle at both
ends.

Chapter 9
Finding the Time

Most women are hard-pressed for time. You could be the mother of a newly born child who needs your full attention. Or you might be a career woman with demanding deadlines and you still need to juggle your duties as a wife.

We live in a fast-paced world. Everybody is running the rat race to be the best rat. There never seems to be enough time, which is a valuable resource. So what do you do?

You improvise. That's what you do.

To put things in perspective, you must realize that there are 24 hours in a day. An hour of exercise is 4% of your daily routine. A 15-minute workout takes up one percent of your day. An eight-minute workout is "half a percent" of your day!

But what can I achieve in 8 minutes? A lot!

Anybody, no matter how busy, can squeeze in 8 minutes. 8 minutes is too much? How about 4 minutes? What?! 4 minutes?

Yes. 4 minutes of Tabata protocol. You can Google it to find out more. The point here is that you can cause a metabolic boost to your body and put it in fat burning mode within 4 minutes and you will be in a fat burning state for hours. Will it be easy? No. But it will be effective.

If you do not have time for one hour long workouts, do quick bursts of 15 minutes or even less. The difference is that the shorter workouts will have to be more intense. However, it will be for a short while only.

There are other ways to make sure you burn more calories. Get yourself a pair of ankle weights and wear them throughout the day.

You will burn more calories when you walk and move. If you're a stay at home mom, get a haversack and add some weight in it. Stow away a phone book or two and put on the haversack.

The added weight will make everything more difficult and you will be burning more calories because of the added resistance.

Invest in a Fitbit so you can monitor your daily step count. Every day, try to increase the amount of steps by 100. Take the stairs rather than the elevator. Walk to the supermarket if you can.

If you're the mother of a newborn, get an infant sling and place your baby in it. Then proceed for a 30-minute walk. Excellent exercise for you and the baby gets a breath of fresh air too.

You may not have enough time. Yet, with a bit of imagination, you can incorporate many little practices and changes in your life to burn more calories. Once you have that done, get a journal and record your hourly activities.

See where your time goes. "Oh look! I'm watching Sex and the City reruns daily!". Ah hah! A time waster right there. Cut it out and spend that 30 minutes exercising. Samantha, you'll benefit more from it than from watching other people try to make out with all the males in New York.

Do whatever you can with whatever time you have. Even if it's only 4 minutes.

Chapter 10
Structuring Your Workouts

One cannot overemphasize the importance of following a good training regimen that not just boosts your stamina but also strengthens and tones your body.

Cardio is a fantastic method for weight loss and calorie burning.

Worldwide, millions of women ONLY concentrate on aerobic exercise. This is a mistake because strength training is crucial for weight loss, too.

The more lean muscle mass your body has, the more calories it burns while at rest.

This practically implies that you will burn fat all day long.

The best way to structure your workout will be to have 3 cardio sessions a week and two resistance training sessions.

The Power of Fasted Cardio

Cardio is extremely effective when done on an empty stomach.

You may have heard that exercising on an empty stomach is great for weight loss. Most people, however, find it difficult to become excited about an intense workout so soon after waking up.

The good news is that it doesn't need to be physically demanding.

It's actually preferable to keep things simple.

One of the best ways to lose weight is to go for a brisk walk first thing in the morning. A short 20 to 30-minute walk is ideal.

You ought to be able to carry on a discussion while moving. You shouldn't be exerting yourself to a point where you're panting and gasping.

We're not aiming for high intensity here.

Your body is fasting when you get up in the morning. Your glycogen levels are low and the food in your body would digest it.

This means that it will force your body to burn fat for fuel while you walk. So, during the 20 to 30 minutes that you're walking, your body is burning its fat stores for fuel.

This is a powerful method, and since it's not strenuous, you can do it daily.

The morning walk will also boost your metabolic rate and you'll burn more calories throughout the day.

If walking isn't your thing, you can swim or ride a stationary bike. Your body will burn fat during moderate-paced cardio exercise, and you'll see the result if you work hard.

You may wish to engage in strength training or a short, high-intensity interval training later in the day. That's perfectly fine because the morning workout is just meant to speed up the fat burning process.

It's an additional technique to help you reach your weight goals faster. This is such an easy method that anyone can do it.

If all you can do is a 10-minute walk, then just do 10 minutes. With time, you can slowly progress to 20 or 30 minutes.

Really, there's no reason to stay for more than 30 minutes.

You will notice a difference in a few weeks if you use this strategy.

Weight training

Many women are afraid that if they lift weights, they will become bulky and muscular like males. This is not the case.

Even man's struggle with gaining muscle. Women who train with weights will look leaner and more defined, but they will not become manly.

You can cast aside all worries about looking like a female bodybuilder.

Bodyweight training such as squats, push-ups, lunges, dips, and pull-ups are great ways to work your muscles and joints.

Exercise your muscles to prevent them from atrophying as you age. Look for exercises that tone your thighs, butt and arms.

These are common problem areas for many women. While cardio will help you shed the fat, strength training will give you the curves and definition that will make you look fit, healthy and radiant.

A short 10 to 15 minute full-body workout done early in the day will work miracles. HIIT is the name for this kind of exercise. Training using High Intensity Intervals.

Here's the kicker. You can even do a HIIT workout in one spot and still sweat like crazy.

Let's examine this exercise routine as an illustration.

Sit-Ups—45 seconds

Burpees—45 seconds

Jump Squats–45 seconds

Push Ups–45 seconds

High Knees–45 seconds

Jumping Jacks–45 seconds

Burpees–45 seconds

Alternating Lung Jumps–45 sec

Sit-ups–45 seconds

Push Ups–45 seconds

You will rest for 15 seconds between each exercise before moving on to the next. You can practice this exercise in a cubicle. It takes up that little space. BUT, most people will not be able to even make it to the 9th exercise.

Why?

Because of the intensity. You need to go as hard as you can go. There is no taking it easy. If all you have is 10 minutes, then it MUST be a hard 10 minutes.

Fortunately, this will just take ten minutes. You'll be in there

'hurt box' during this time, but you need to keep telling yourself…

"It's only 10 minutes! I can do this."

It's possible to complete an exercise regimen during a commercial break. It's that fast. If you do this workout early in the day, your body will be in fat burning mode throughout the day because of the intensity.

It induces what it means to post-exercise oxygen utilization in your body. It means that for 10 or even 14 hours after your workout, your body will continue to burn calories at a higher rate.

It's amazing what just 10 minutes can do.

You do it early in the day because your metabolism drops once you go to bed. By completing your training early in the day, you'll get maximum rewards.

It's also worth noting that it's best that you make these short workouts full body workouts. Do compound movements such as squats, jumps, push ups, etc.

By recruiting as many muscles in your body, make sure your workout engages the whole body.

Don't just try to wing it with simple exercises such as dumbbell curls and call it a day. All you have is 10 minutes. You have to make it count.

Within a month, just three of these quick workouts a week will completely change your body. Go ahead and give them a try. The results will amaze you.

Do remember to have 2 rest days a week. You can split them up or you can have both days back to back. It's really up to you.

Take a weekly break to allow your muscles and central nervous system to heal. Your body will grow weary and agitated if you push yourself too hard without taking breaks.

It's possible that you'll reach a weight loss plateau, after which there won't be any more weight reduction regardless of your efforts.

After that, take four or five days off to rest. This will slow your progress down, and you might even put on weight.

Take a 2 day break every week.

Find the best cardio and resistance training programs by doing web research.

Challenge your body with different workouts. It won't take long for you to get stronger and more slender.

Chapter 11
Putting the Fun In It

Make your exercise sessions fun. Find a workout buddy if you need one.

Don't do the same workouts daily. Monotony can discourage even the most enthusiastic woman.

Try something new, like yoga at the gym or kickboxing.

You could try rock-climbing too!

Feel like dancing? Watch Shaun T's exercise videos and give them a try.

The key here is to keep moving. Watch Shaun T's exercise videos and give them a try.

Here, it's important to stay moving.
Whatever you do, your calorie deficit will
result in weight loss.

The goal of the exercise is to expedite the
procedure.

Do whatever you like. Cycling, running,
swimming.

What matters is that you MOVE daily. The
root cause of obesity is a sedentary lifestyle.

Keep moving and keep it fun.

Chapter 12
Dealing with Slip-Ups

It's going to happen. Sooner or later it definitely is going to happen. "What's going to happen?" you ask.

You're going to slip up on your diet and eat something you know you shouldn't or you may not do a workout that you know you should.

It happens to almost all of us. Whether you succeed or fail horribly in your weight loss quest depends entirely on how you handle your mistakes moving forward.

Let's start by discussing diet errors. When you go on a weight loss journey, it usually involves eating less than you're accustomed to, in order to create a caloric deficit. You'll also need to focus on eating foods that are healthy and wholesome while avoiding processed and junk food.

However, the body is already used to eating without much thought and you're probably addicted to processed and junk food without even realizing it. Millions of people are, and when they try to ditch these unhealthy foods, they get cravings and mood swings.

The key point is to make the changes gradual. Only aim for a 500-calorie deficit daily. This is a reasonable quantity, so you won't get hunger pangs.

You may feel a little peckish but it will be manageable. If you cut your calories too drastically, you will be feeling hungry all the time and this is sheer mental and physical torture.

Changing your foods overnight causes the same problem. Your body is not used to it. The goal is to progressively cut back on unhealthy food intake and swap it out for healthier options.

If you typically drink three soda cans every day, try cutting it down to two for a week, then just one can and finally give up the soda habit entirely. Don't give up soda all at once.

Problems arise when people try to do too much too soon. They make things so challenging that compliance becomes a nightmare. People aim for perfection.

Eventually, they give in to temptation and devour a bag of cookies or a greasy cheeseburger and fries after losing the internal struggle to control themselves.

They believe they have failed and feel guilty when it occurs. Then, they give up on their goal and throw in the towel, believing that they are destined to be overweight. Millions of individuals experience this, which is why so many give up.

When you make a mistake, the first thing to recognize is that you only made one. You have not failed yet. You only fail when you give up. If you accidentally dropped your mobile phone, wouldn't you quickly pick it up, dust it off, and keep it safely?

Surely you wouldn't keep dropping it and smashing it because of the first accident.

Likewise, own up to your mistakes and move forward. Make a promise to yourself that you will watch what you consume. Let go of your strict diet and give yourself some leeway, all the while keeping your calorie deficit intact. Avoid depriving yourself too quickly of too much.

You should think the same way about your workouts. Make sure you work out the following day if you are unable to do so today. Never skip more than three consecutive workouts; if you do, you'll easily veer off course and find it extremely difficult to get back on track.

If you dread exercising, you're either pushing yourself too hard or you're engaged in an activity that you have no interest in.

Exercise is meant to boost your metabolic rate and increase fat burning. Your diet and caloric deficit are what really matters when it comes to fat loss.

Dietary errors and skipped workouts are not fatalities, and your weight loss efforts shouldn't come to an end because of them.

It's a trip, so occasionally getting lost along the road is unavoidable. You will succeed if you don't give up and endure through your obstacles. Most people virtually always accomplish their goals in this way. Keep going forward and keep your chin up.

Chapter 13
Taking Time to Smell the Roses

There will be moments when you want to give up completely. This is typical.
All you have to do is unwind and like the procedure. Accept a pound of weight loss as success. Next week, you can shed even more weight.
It's important to have faith in your ability to succeed and to maintain an optimistic outlook.
Remain detached from your weight. Retain the calorie deficit, exercise, hydrate well, get enough rest, enjoy your exercise, and relax. You will reach your goal. Watch a movie or a comedy to destress. Go on a vacation, but don't throw your diet away.
Always keep your chin up and keep going in the future. You'll arrive at your desired location if you can visualize it.

Chapter 14
Getting There and Staying There

Most women who lose weight often gain it back after a while. Even people on TV shows such as The Biggest Loser gained all the fat they all once the show ended.
You have to alter your way of life if you want to stay thin.
Whatever you learn in this book, you will need to put into practice from now on.

You will need to consume your calories at a maintenance level once you have reached your optimum weight. This will guarantee that you don't put on or lose additional weight.
To stay in shape, keep up your current fitness regimen.

You'll need to be alert. A rolling stone doesn't collect moss. so you'll have to persevere.

Conclusion

Well, you've reached the end of the book.

If you follow what was stated in here without giving up, you will reach the body you desire.

Remain persistent. Give up if you're sick of beginning over.

You're capable of it.

Millions of women have lost weight and managed to keep it off. You can make it happen as well if others can.

All the best in your weight loss journey.